DANCE THERAPY FOR EMOTIONAL EXPRESSION

Complete Guide To Explore The Healing Power Of Dance Therapy, Understand Its Techniques, And Embrace Emotional Expression In Every Step

WILFREDO CARSON

INTRODUCTION

Dance Therapy, a distinct and emerging form of expressive arts therapy, has a substantial impact on emotional well-being and psychological rehabilitation. Dance therapy, founded on the premise that the body and mind are inextricably linked, uses the power of movement and creative expression to promote emotional, mental, and physical well-being. This introduction discusses the history of dance therapy, the goal and scope of the book, and the significance of emotional expression in treatment.

Background on Dance Therapy

Dance therapy, also known as dance movement therapy (DMT), arose in the mid-twentieth century as a therapeutic technique that uses movement and dance to help people overcome emotional, cognitive, and physical issues. Dance therapy originated with significant pioneers such as Marian Chace and Rudolf Laban, who recognized the tremendous impact of movement on psychological well-being.

Chace, regarded as the father of dance therapy, presented the concept of employing dance as a kind of psychotherapy in the 1940s, opening the way for the establishment of a distinct therapeutic profession.

Dance therapy has evolved, drawing on principles from psychology, neuroscience, and other dance genres. It is used in a wide range of contexts, including mental health facilities, schools, community centers, and private offices. Dance therapists use dance to help people explore and express their feelings.

They have a thorough understanding of both movement and psychology.

The therapy method consists of movement observation, verbal communication, and the establishment of a secure and supportive environment in which clients can freely express themselves.

Goals and Purpose of the Book

The goal of this book is to explore the various components of dance therapy for emotional expression. The book attempts to provide a full grasp of dance therapy's theoretical foundations, practical applications, and case studies. It investigates the various uses of dance therapy across demographics, age ranges, and cultural contexts, offering light on its adaptability and inclusiveness.

The book explores essential themes in dance therapy, such as the therapeutic connection, movement analysis, symbolism, and the integration of different therapeutic methods.

It also discusses the obstacles and ethical issues involved in the practice of dance therapy, emphasizing the need for cultural sensitivity and the necessity for continued study to improve the efficacy of this therapeutic technique.

The book also emphasizes the significance of dance therapy in improving emotional intelligence, resilience, and overall well-being.

Importance of Emotional Expression in Therapy.

Emotional expressiveness is an essential component of the human experience, influencing mental health and overall well-being. In therapy, the ability to express and process emotions is critical to healing and personal development. Emotional expression enables people to release pent-up emotions, gain insight into their inner world, and create stronger coping methods.

In this section, we will look at the importance of emotional expression in treatment and how dance therapy specifically aids this process.

Emotions, whether pleasant or negative, are fundamental to the human experience. Suppressing or denying emotions can result in a variety of psychological and physical problems, including anxiety, despair, and somatic symptoms.

Traditional talk treatments have long acknowledged the significance of verbal expression in resolving emotions. However, dance therapy broadens the therapeutic toolkit by including nonverbal modes of communication through movement.

Dance therapy offers a unique way for people to communicate emotions that might be difficult to define properly. Movement allows patients to access and articulate emotions hidden in their bodies, allowing for a more holistic and embodied approach to treatment.

The body acts as a canvas for emotional expression, and dance therapists are taught to monitor and interpret nonverbal signs in their clients' movements.

Furthermore, dance therapy fosters a mind-body connection, recognizing that emotions are not limited to the head but can also appear in the body.

Dance allows people to explore and relieve stress, trauma, and unspoken sentiments.

This holistic approach helps to provide a more comprehensive therapeutic experience by addressing both the cognitive and physical aspects of emotional expression.

In addition to providing a nonverbal medium for expression, dancing therapy promotes creativity and self-discovery.

Individuals who engage in movement and dance may discover and explore feelings that they were previously unaware of.

The symbolic nature of dance movements gives a rich and subtle language for expressing complicated emotional states, allowing for a better knowledge of oneself.

Furthermore, dance therapy is naturally inclusive, accepting a wide range of ethnic expressions and personal preferences. Movement is a universal means of expression, as opposed to verbal communication, which might be limited by language obstacles or personal inhibitions.

This universality makes dance therapy accessible to people of all ages, ethnicities, and abilities, fostering inclusivity in the therapeutic process.

The significance of emotional expression in treatment cannot be emphasized, and dance therapy emerges as a dynamic and successful modality for promoting such expression. Dance therapy is a holistic approach to emotional well-being by using movement and creativity, addressing the interconnectedness of the mind and body.

The following sections of this book will go into greater detail on the theoretical foundations, practical applications, and case studies that demonstrate dance therapy's transforming capacity for emotional expression.

CHAPTER 1
UNDERSTANDING DANCE THERAPY

Definition and Concepts of Dance Therapy:

Dance therapy, often known as dance movement therapy (DMT), is a type of expressive therapy that uses movement and dance to improve emotional, mental, and physical health. It is founded on the notion that the mind and body are inextricably linked and that through deliberate movement, people can explore, express, and process their feelings. Dance therapy extends beyond standard verbal communication, providing a unique opportunity for self-discovery and healing. Practitioners, who are often trained in both dance and psychotherapy, lead sessions that encourage clients to utilize movement to express themselves and explore their emotions.

Historical Evolution of Dance as Therapy:

dancing therapy has its roots in ancient civilizations, where dancing was an important aspect of ceremonies and therapeutic procedures. However, the formalization of dance therapy as a therapeutic strategy occurred in the twentieth century. Marian Chace and Rudolf Laban were pioneers in developing and promoting dance therapy.

In the early 1940s, Chace began bringing movement into psychiatric settings, establishing the framework for dance's inclusion into conventional mental health procedures. Over the years, the field has changed, including new approaches and adapting to varied cultural contexts.

Theoretical Frameworks for Dance Therapy

Psychodynamic Approach:

The psychodynamic approach in dance therapy is based on psychoanalytic theories and stresses the investigation of the unconscious mind via movement. Practitioners who use this method believe that movement patterns and expressions can disclose buried emotions and unsolved issues. Individuals can tap into their unconscious through dance, allowing them to uncover repressed feelings and experiences. The therapist's goal is to help clients grasp and integrate these disclosures, promoting self-awareness and emotional healing.

Humanistic approach:

The humanistic approach to dance therapy is based on the concept that humans have the potential for self-actualization and personal progress. It is consistent with Carl Rogers' person-centered therapy, which emphasizes empathy, unconditional positive regard, and sincerity. The humanistic approach to dance therapy allows people to express themselves authentically via movement. The therapist fosters a supportive environment in which people feel free to express their emotions without fear of being judged, so encouraging self-discovery and empowerment.

<u>Cognitive-behavioural Approach:</u>

The cognitive-behavioural approach to dance therapy incorporates elements from cognitive-behavioural therapy (CBT), with a focus on the link between thoughts, feelings, and behaviors. In this approach, movement is used to detect and change dysfunctional cognitive processes and behaviors.

Dance therapists who use this technique work with clients to identify negative thought patterns in their movement, providing possibilities for cognitive restructuring and behaviour modification. This technique seeks to improve emotional well-being by encouraging beneficial cognitive and behavioural changes via dancing.

<u>Benefits of Dance Therapy for Emotional Wellbeing:</u>

Dance therapy has numerous benefits to mental well-being, making it an effective therapeutic method in a variety of contexts. One notable advantage is its capacity to provide a nonverbal channel for emotional expression.

Many people struggle to describe their emotions verbally, and dance therapy provides an alternate form of communication. Clients can use movement to communicate complex emotions, release pent-up feelings, and gain insight into their emotional states.

Dance therapy also encourages people to connect with their bodies and emotions, which helps them become more aware of themselves. Clients can tune into physiological sensations by mindfully exploring movement patterns, allowing them to have a better understanding of their emotions. This increased self-awareness is an important step towards emotional regulation and personal development.

Furthermore, dancing therapy can be particularly effective in treating trauma and PTSD.

Traumatic events frequently emerge in the body, and dance therapy offers a safe environment for people to process and express trauma-related emotions via movement. The planned yet flexible nature of dance therapy sessions allows for gradual exposure and healing, assisting individuals on their path to recovery.

Another major benefit of dance therapy is its ability to improve interpersonal skills and foster social ties. Group dance therapy sessions establish a social environment in which people can express themselves through movement, fostering a sense of connection and belonging. This social dimension promotes emotional well-being by alleviating emotions of isolation and loneliness.

Furthermore, the physical part of dance therapy promotes emotional well-being. Movement produces endorphins, the body's natural mood boosters, which promote a pleasant emotional state. Regular participation in dance therapy has been associated with lower levels of despair and anxiety, suggesting its potential as a supplemental intervention in mental health care.

Dance therapy takes a holistic approach to emotional well-being, combining movement, self-expression, and therapeutic ideas. Its historical history, various theoretical frameworks, and countless benefits highlight its importance as a useful treatment technique. Dance therapy, whether employed in individual or group settings, can provide significant emotional insights and transforming experiences for anyone looking to improve their emotional health and overall well-being.

CHAPTER 2
THE CONNECTION BETWEEN DANCE AND EMOTIONS

Dance therapy, a type of expressive arts therapy, is based on the complex interplay between dance and emotions. Dancing is a wonderful tool for people to connect with and express their feelings in a nonverbal way.

In this therapeutic environment, movement serves as a medium for exploring and communicating feelings. Dance allows people to dig into their deepest feelings, bridging language barriers and providing an alternate form of emotional expression. The connection between dance and emotions stems from the significant effect that physical movement has on the human psyche.

<u>How Movement Influences Emotions:</u>

Exploring how movement affects emotions is an important part of understanding dance's therapeutic usefulness. Physical movement, particularly in the setting of dance therapy, is thought to increase the release of neurotransmitters and endorphins in the brain. This biological response regulates mood and emotional well-being. Individuals who engage in focused and guided movement might gain a greater sense of self-awareness, helping them to better connect with and process their emotions. Furthermore, the rhythmic and regulated pattern of dance movements can produce a state of flow, encouraging mindfulness and presence, which aids in emotional regulation.

Neuroscientific Foundations of Dance and Emotional Expression:

The neuroscientific basis of dance and emotional expression dives into the complex interplay of brain functions, neuronal connections, and physiological responses to dance. Neuroscientific study has shown that dancing engages a variety of brain regions, including those responsible for motor control, emotion processing, and memory.

Dance promotes pleasure and emotional well-being by releasing neurotransmitters such as dopamine and serotonin. Furthermore, the repetitive and synchronized movements involved in dance may improve neuroplasticity, affecting the brain's ability to adapt and restructure itself. Understanding the neuroscientific foundations of dance offers vital insights into how this type of treatment might improve emotional expressiveness and mental health.

Cultural Perspectives on Dance and Emotional Release.

Cultural perspectives on dance and emotional release emphasize the diversity of dance styles seen in various countries, as well as the particular manner in which they allow emotional outpouring. The cultural environment has a tremendous impact on the symbolism, rituals, and emotional connotations linked with dancing. In certain cultures, dance is a community activity that fosters a sense of belonging and shared emotional experiences. In other cases, dance may be strongly established in spiritual or religious activities, providing a means for people to communicate with higher forces or ancestral spirits. Exploring the cultural components of dance in the context of emotional release emphasizes the significance of acknowledging and respecting many points of view on the therapeutic usefulness of movement and expression. This cultural awareness is critical to the effectiveness of dance therapy in addressing emotional well-being on a worldwide scale.

Dance therapy works at the crossroads of movement and emotional expression, making use of the natural connection between the two to enhance psychological well-being. Understanding how movement impacts emotions, investigating the neuroscientific basis of dance, and appreciating cultural perspectives on emotional release through dance all contribute to a more complete understanding of the therapeutic mechanisms at play. As a comprehensive approach to mental health, dance therapy provides a complex and culturally sensitive framework for people to explore, analyze, and express their feelings in ways that go beyond verbal communication.

CHAPTER 3
PRINCIPLES AND TECHNIQUES IN DANCE THERAPY

Setting Up a Therapeutic Dance Environment:

Creating a therapeutic dancing setting is essential to the practice of dance therapy for emotional expression. This idea comprises both the physical and emotional areas in which the therapeutic process occurs. The therapist is responsible for creating a safe, nonjudgmental, and supportive environment that enables self-expression. The physical environment, including the dance studio or treatment room, must be favourable to movement and free expression. Additionally, lighting, music, and space organization all contribute to the overall environment. Therapists strive to create a setting that promotes trust and openness, allowing clients to express their feelings via movement. This part of dance therapy is consistent with the larger ideas of person-centered therapy, emphasizing the role of the therapeutic interaction and environment in supporting emotional healing and self-discovery.

Embodied Awareness and Mindfulness in Dance.

Dance therapy relies heavily on embodied awareness and mindfulness for emotional expression. In this context, embodiment refers to the relationship between the mind and the body, stressing a person's awareness of their bodily sensations, movements, and feelings. Mindfulness, based on contemplative practices, entails being fully present in the present moment without judgment.

Using these ideas in dance therapy improves self-awareness and emotional regulation. Therapists assist clients in exploring their sensations, breath, and movement patterns, resulting in a better understanding of their emotional experiences. Individuals who engage in mindful movement might acquire a greater awareness of their bodies, resulting in increased self-compassion and emotional understanding. This blending of embodiment and mindfulness is consistent with holistic approaches to mental health, which recognize the interdependence of the mind and body in the treatment process.

Improvisation and the Creative Movement:

Dance therapy incorporates the concepts of improvisation and creative movement, which provide a dynamic and expressive outlet for emotional exploration.

Improvisation entails spontaneous, unplanned movement, which allows people to overcome cognitive filters and connect directly with their emotions. Therapists urge clients to trust their instincts, fostering authenticity and self-discovery. The creative movement goes beyond improvisation, integrating organized but inventive activities to elicit specific feelings or ideas. This strategy enables people to discuss and process complicated emotions that may be difficult to express verbally.

Dance therapy uses improvisation and creative movement to serve as a vehicle for symbolic expression, allowing clients to externalize and make sense of their internal reality. This is consistent with ideas emphasizing the importance of nonverbal communication and symbolic representation in understanding and processing emotions.

<u>Guided Movement Exploration:</u>

Guided movement exploration is a core technique in dance therapy in which the therapist gives clients organized cues or themes to explore via movement. This style combines elements of improvisation and creative movement while providing a more concentrated concentration. Therapists can help clients explore certain emotions, memories, or interpersonal dynamics through movement. The regulated aspect of guided movement exploration allows participants to deal with their emotions in a supportive and contained environment. It provides a mix of spontaneity and thoughtfulness, resulting in a stronger connection to one's emotional landscape. This technique is especially useful for people who may struggle with the open-ended nature of improvisation, as it provides a scaffolded approach to emotional expression through movement.

Integrating Music into Dance Therapy:

The incorporation of music into dance therapy enhances the emotional and therapeutic effects of movement. Music is a strong instrument for evoking emotions, setting the tone, and enhancing the sensory experience. Therapists carefully choose music based on the therapeutic goals and emotional states they want to explore with their clients. The rhythm, tempo, and melody of music can impact the pace and intensity of movement, resulting in a dynamic and expressive medium. The use of music in dance therapy is consistent with music therapy theories, which emphasize the connectivity of music and emotions. It adds complexity to the therapy process by engaging both the aural and tactile senses. Dance therapists can create a multisensory experience by using music intentionally, which deepens emotional expression, aids emotional regulation, and improves the session's overall therapeutic impact.

CHAPTER 4
ASSESSING EMOTIONAL STATES THROUGH MOVEMENT

Observation and analysis of movement:

Observation and study of movement are fundamental components of dance therapy for emotional expression. Movement serves as a nonverbal language that expresses a person's emotional state, giving therapists a unique way to analyze and comprehend their clients. Therapists assess individuals' movement quality, intensity, and patterns through close observation. Various components of movement, such as posture, rhythm, and gesture, provide important insights into emotional states. For example, stiff and constricted movements may signify emotional anguish, whereas fluid and expansive movements may reflect a sense of liberation and release. The therapist's ability to recognize these distinctions allows for a more sophisticated comprehension of the client's emotional landscape. This procedure is based on a holistic approach that takes into account the connection of mind and body, emphasizing the interdependence of emotional and physical well-being.

Developing Individualized Dance Therapy Plans:

The creation of personalized dance therapy programs is an essential component of using dance as a therapeutic tool for emotional expression. Each person has a distinct mix of emotional experiences, traumas, and coping strategies, necessitating a tailored approach to dance therapy.

Therapists collaborate with their clients to define specific emotional goals and adjust interventions accordingly.

The therapeutic dance plans include a wide range of movement-based activities such as improvisation, guided movement exploration, and planned sequences. These plans incorporate client-centered therapy ideas and are flexible and adjustable to meet the individual's changing emotional requirements. A thorough assessment of the client's emotional states guides the selection of appropriate dance interventions, resulting in a therapeutic process that is both successful and suited to the client's unique emotional journey.

<u>Case Studies Demonstrating Emotional Expression Assessment:</u>

Case studies are invaluable for understanding the actual use of dance therapy in measuring emotional expression.

These real-life examples demonstrate the various ways in which people use movement to express and process their emotions. Through in-depth examination of individual instances, therapists and researchers develop a better grasp of the complexities of emotional expression assessment in dance therapy.

Case studies enable the evaluation of the efficacy of various therapeutic modalities, giving insight into the complexities of emotional states and the transformational power of dance. These narratives not only add to the field's current body of research but also provide inspiration and instruction for practitioners looking to improve their skills in emotional expression evaluation through movement.

Finally, case studies highlight the dynamic and individualized aspect of dance therapy, emphasizing its ability to address a wide range of emotional difficulties.

In summary, assessing emotional states through movement in dance therapy is a multidimensional process that includes movement observation and analysis, the construction of specific therapeutic programs, and case study examination. Therapists learn about their clients' emotional experiences by deciphering the nonverbal language of movement. The establishment of personalized therapy programs guarantees that therapies are tailored to each individual's specific emotional requirements. Case studies add to our understanding of emotional expression assessment in dance therapy by demonstrating its practical application.

Together, these ideas add to the growing discipline of dance therapy, emphasizing its effectiveness in promoting emotional expression and well-being.

CHAPTER 5
APPLICATIONS OF DANCE THERAPY

Dance therapy, also known as dance movement therapy (DMT), is a comprehensive approach to healing that uses movement and dance to promote emotional, physical, and mental well-being. This treatment method has found applications in a variety of fields, contributing to the general improvement of people's lives. This section delves into the various applications of dance therapy in mental health, physical rehabilitation, and education contexts.

Dance Therapy for Mental Health.

Dance therapy has proven to be an effective intervention in the field of mental health, treating a wide range of emotional difficulties that individuals may confront. One notable area is the treatment of anxiety and stress. Dance's rhythmic and expressive character allows people to relieve tension and explore their feelings via movement. Participants learn to control their breathing, manage stress, and build coping techniques through controlled sessions.

The nonverbal nature of dance therapy is very effective for people who struggle to express their emotions vocally.

Dance therapy can help people with depression reconnect with their bodies and emotions. The physical exertion inherent in dance promotes the release of endorphins, the body's natural mood boosters. Furthermore, dance's creative expression allows individuals to externalize and process their internal challenges, promoting empowerment and self-awareness.

Addressing trauma is another important part of dance therapy in mental health. Traumatic experiences frequently leave imprints on both the mind and the body, and typical talk therapies may be ineffective in treating the physical impacts of trauma.

Dance therapy is a non-intrusive way for people to examine and remove trauma from their bodies. The guided movements and therapeutic relationship formed with the dance therapist provide a safe environment for people to gradually process and integrate their painful experiences.

<u>Dance Therapy for Physical Rehab</u>

Aside from its effects on mental health, dance therapy has shown promise in the domain of physical rehabilitation.

Dance therapy treats chronic pain by using movement to increase body awareness and improve movement quality.

The mind-body connection inherent in dancing enables individuals to detect and correct movement habits that may be contributing to their pain.

Individuals can benefit from the incorporation of dance into rehabilitation programs by reducing pain and increasing functionality, improving overall wellness.

Dance therapy can also help with motor skill improvement in physical rehabilitation. Whether people are healing from neurological illnesses like strokes or dealing with developmental issues, dancing therapy offers a dynamic and engaging platform for improving motor skills.

Dance requires intentional movements, which help people develop their coordination, balance, and spatial awareness. In addition to the physical benefits, dance provides sensory and emotional experiences that aid in the healing process.

<u>Dance Therapy in Educational Settings</u>

Dance therapy is emerging as an effective technique in educational settings to meet varied learning demands and promote holistic development.

Dance therapy can help schools improve the social and emotional well-being of their children. One of its primary advantages is its capacity to accommodate varied learning styles and preferences, resulting in an inclusive and adaptive therapeutic approach.

Dance therapy has had a significant influence on people with a variety of cognitive and developmental difficulties, particularly in special education settings.

Dance's nonverbal and tactile nature facilitates communication across language boundaries, providing a medium of expression for those who struggle with verbal communication.

In special education, dancing therapy serves as a creative outlet for students of various abilities, encouraging a sense of accomplishment and self-esteem.

Dance therapy's applications in mental health, physical rehabilitation, and education demonstrate its adaptability as a therapeutic modality.

Its ability to treat a wide range of needs and enhance overall well-being emphasizes the importance of incorporating movement and dance into a broader range of therapeutic therapies.

CHAPTER 6
CULTURAL CONSIDERATIONS IN DANCE THERAPY

variety in Dance Forms: Exploring cultural variety within dance therapy is critical to understanding the rich tapestry of expressive movement throughout societies. Different nations have unique dance forms that are strongly ingrained in their traditions, history, and social behaviors. Recognizing and embracing diversity in dance therapy is critical for giving appropriate emotional expression outlets to people from all backgrounds. For example, classical dance forms such as Bharatanatyam in India and Flamenco in Spain have distinct emotional nuances and symbolism that can be used in therapeutic contexts.

Understanding the cultural relevance of various dance forms enables therapists to develop therapies that align with their clients' cultural identities, thus increasing the therapeutic benefit of the practice.

Cross-Cultural Approaches to Emotional Expression: Due to the worldwide character of dance therapy, practitioners must use cross-cultural approaches that transcend geographical and societal borders.

This entails not just embracing many dance traditions, but also acknowledging the universality of certain emotional responses conveyed through movement. While cultural differences enrich dance therapy, common strands of human experience unite people around the world. Exploring these connections enables the development of cross-cultural therapies that promote emotional expressiveness regardless of cultural origin. This technique encourages inclusivity and allows therapists to establish a secure and supportive environment in which clients can participate in the therapy process, supporting emotional well-being in a cross-cultural setting.

Addressing Cultural Sensitivity in Dance Therapy: Cultural sensitivity is a fundamental principle of dance therapy that drives ethical and effective treatments. This requires a sophisticated awareness of cultural norms, values, and beliefs to guarantee that dance therapy is respectful and inclusive. Therapists must avoid the problems of cultural appropriation and misinterpretation while emphasizing the significance of authenticity in incorporating cultural elements into therapeutic methods. Furthermore, the recognition of power dynamics within the therapeutic interaction is critical, as therapists must be aware of the possible impact of their cultural prejudices on the therapeutic process. Dance therapists who prioritize cultural sensitivity can establish a therapeutic atmosphere that values variety, encourages emotional expression, and fosters a sense of cultural safety for clients.

These three interconnected concepts highlight the importance of cultural considerations in the field of dance therapy, emphasizing the need for therapists to navigate the complex interplay of cultural diversity, cross-cultural approaches, and cultural sensitivity to improve the efficacy and ethicality of their practice.

CHAPTER 7
PROFESSIONAL PRACTICES AND ETHICS

The area of dance therapy is distinguished by a dedication to upholding high professional standards and ethical principles.

The credentials and training of dance therapists is an important factor in assuring the effectiveness and safety of the practice.

These professionals receive extensive education and training to gain the required skills and expertise for dealing with diverse groups. Dance therapists' qualifications often include academic education, supervised clinical practice, and continued professional development. This comprehensive program prepares therapists to traverse the complicated convergence of movement, psychology, and psychotherapy.

Ethical considerations are the foundation of dance therapy practice. Practitioners in this industry must follow a code of ethics that governs their dealings with clients, coworkers, and the larger community. Dance therapy places a high value on ethical concepts such as secrecy, autonomy, and cultural sensitivity. Maintaining confidentiality is especially important given the sensitive and frequently vulnerable nature of the therapy process. Dance therapists must strike a difficult balance between providing a safe environment for expression and maintaining their clients' privacy and dignity.

Furthermore, collaboration with other healthcare specialists is an important part of dance therapy. Individuals seeking therapeutic assistance benefit from interdisciplinary collaboration, which provides holistic and integrated care. Dance therapists frequently collaborate with psychologists, psychiatrists, physical therapists, and other healthcare specialists to provide a holistic approach to rehabilitation. This partnership allows for more detailed knowledge of the client's requirements and the synergistic integration of multiple therapy modalities.

Qualifications and Training for Dance Therapists

Dance therapists' qualifications and training are essential components that contribute to their professional competence and effectiveness. Individuals who want to become dance therapists often acquire a master's degree in dance/movement therapy or a comparable subject. This formal education gives therapists a solid basis in both dance and psychology, preparing them to incorporate movement into therapeutic interactions.

Dance therapy programs address a wide range of topics, including dance improvisation, movement psychology, clinical assessment, and therapeutic ethics. Supervised clinical practice is an important part of the training process, allowing prospective dance therapists to apply theoretical knowledge in real-world therapy settings. This hands-on experience, guided by professional supervisors, allows therapists to enhance clinical skills, acquire confidence, and fine-tune their approach to working with varied groups.

Dance therapy also emphasizes continual professional development. Therapists are urged to attend workshops, conferences, and continuing education to stay current on the most recent research, therapeutic approaches, and ethical requirements. This dedication to lifelong learning guarantees that dance therapists are always knowledgeable and adaptable in their profession, constantly improving the level of care they deliver to their clients.

Ethical Considerations for Dance Therapy

Ethical issues are critical in guiding dance therapists' behavior and ensuring their clients' well-being. Confidentiality is one of the most essential ethical considerations in dance therapy. Dance therapists are entrusted with sensitive and personal information during the therapy process, and keeping this information private is critical to establishing trust and providing a secure therapeutic environment. Clients require assurance that their personal information will be treated with the highest confidentiality.

Respect for autonomy is another essential component of ethical dance therapy practice. This principle recognizes the autonomy and self-determination of clients during the therapeutic process. Dance therapists collaborate with clients, respecting their decisions and preferences while helping them through the discovery of dance as a form of emotional expression. Respecting autonomy also entails getting clients' informed permission, which ensures they are completely aware of the therapy process and any potential dangers or advantages.

Cultural sensitivity is an ethical obligation in dance therapy, which recognizes and respects clients' different cultural backgrounds. Therapists must be sensitive to cultural differences that can influence movement expression and perception. Recognizing and respecting cultural variety enhances dance therapy's inclusion, making it accessible and meaningful to people from many cultural, ethnic, and socioeconomic backgrounds.

Additionally, ethical considerations include professional boundaries. Dance therapists must create clear and acceptable boundaries with clients to maintain the therapeutic relationship's integrity. This involves avoiding dual partnerships, in which therapists play numerous roles with clients outside of the therapy setting, to avoid conflicts of interest and potential injury.

Collaboration with Other Healthcare Professionals.

Collaboration with other healthcare specialists is essential for providing complete and integrated care in the field of dance therapy. Dance therapists regularly participate in interdisciplinary collaboration, recognizing that clients seeking treatment may have complex needs. This collaborative method entails working with professionals from a variety of healthcare disciplines, such as psychology, psychiatry, physical therapy, and occupational therapy.

Dance therapists, in collaboration with psychologists and psychiatrists, bring a unique viewpoint to the understanding and treatment of mental health concerns. Movement and dance can be effective tools for emotional expression and self-discovery, supplementing typical talk therapy techniques. Collaboration with mental health specialists includes coordinated case discussions, joint treatment planning, and a comprehensive approach to addressing clients' psychological well-being.

Physical therapists frequently interact with dance therapists in circumstances when movement and physical health are inextricably linked. Dance therapy combined with physical therapy can be very effective for people who suffer from chronic pain, motor coordination difficulties, or neurological issues.

The combined knowledge of dance and physical therapists enables a comprehensive approach that addresses both the physical and emotional aspects of a client's well-being.

Furthermore, contact with occupational therapists is necessary in the framework of dance therapy. Occupational therapists assist people engage in meaningful activities and daily duties. Dance therapists, in partnership with occupational therapists, can create therapies that support clients' goals, improve functional abilities, and increase overall well-being.

Interdisciplinary teamwork benefits clients while also enriching the professional growth of dance therapists. Exposure to other perspectives and experiences broadens the therapeutic toolset, allowing dance therapists to tailor their methods to clients' requirements. This collaborative paradigm shows dance therapy's holistic approach and ability to address the complex interplay of physical, emotional, and psychological well-being.

CHAPTER 8
CASE STUDIES.

Case Study 1: Overcoming Trauma with Dance

In the field of dance therapy, the use of movement and expression has a transforming potential for people living with trauma.

Case Study 1 dives into the use of dance therapy as a means of overcoming trauma. Trauma can emerge in a variety of ways, leaving individuals with emotional scars that traditional therapeutic methods may fail to address fully. Dance therapy, which focuses on nonverbal communication and embodiment, offers a unique way for people to process and release traumatic experiences. The case study delves into the path of a client who has experienced tremendous trauma and how dance therapy aided their healing process. The case study provides light on the varied ways in which dance therapy can aid in the cathartic discharge of trauma while also boosting emotional well-being and resilience.

Case Study 2: Building Emotional Resilience in Adolescents

Adolescence is a time of emotional upheaval and identity formation, making it an important moment for therapies that promote emotional resilience. Case Study 2 looks at how dance therapy can help adolescents improve their emotional resilience. The study investigates the relationship between dance, self-expression, and emotional regulation in the setting of teenage development. Dance therapy's embodied aspect can help adolescents navigate identity, societal expectations, and peer dynamics. The case study examines various dance interventions and therapy strategies to shed light on the role of dance in increasing emotional awareness and regulation in teenagers. It investigates the possible long-term influence on emotional resilience, offering insights into how dance therapy might be integrated into a wider range of mental health therapies for this population.

Case Study 3: Implementing Dance Therapy in a Mental Health Program

pg. 63

The third case study focuses on the systemic integration of dance therapy into a comprehensive mental health program. Mental health programs frequently seek out several approaches to address the multidimensional character of emotional well-being. Case Study 3 looks at the process and results of including dance therapy as a key component of a mental health project. The study dives into logistics, collaboration between mental health specialists and dance therapists, and the influence on program participants. This case study investigates the subtle dynamics of bringing dance therapy into a larger mental health framework. This encompasses program design, participant involvement, and the overall efficacy of an integrated approach to promoting emotional expression and well-being on a larger scale.

CONCLUSION

The three case studies demonstrate the diverse and transformative character of dance therapy in promoting emotional expression and well-being. The therapeutic efficacy of dance in overcoming trauma, improving emotional resilience in teenagers, and incorporating dance therapy into mental health programs demonstrates its adaptability as a potent therapeutic tool. The case studies demonstrate that dance therapy makes a distinctive and valuable addition to the field of mental health. Its emphasis on embodied expression, nonverbal communication, and mind-body integration offers a comprehensive approach to emotional recovery. The case studies' conclusions underline the importance of a comprehensive understanding of dance therapy as a dynamic and changeable solution.

The first case study highlights dance therapy's promise in trauma treatment, demonstrating how movement and expression can be used to relieve deeply ingrained emotional traumas. By investigating specific dance moves and therapeutic approaches used, it becomes clear that dance therapy provides individuals with a safe and non-intrusive environment in which to process and overcome traumatic events. This not only helps with emotional release but also promotes the development of coping strategies and resilience.

Moving on to the second case study, the emphasis changes to the adolescent demographic, which frequently deals with the challenges of identity development and emotional regulation.

The case study highlights the importance of dance therapy in giving adolescents a way to express themselves genuinely. By evaluating specific dance therapies suited to this demographic's developmental needs, the study sheds light on how dance therapy might help with emotional awareness, regulation, and, ultimately, resilience.

 It emphasizes the possibilities of incorporating dance therapy into school and community contexts to improve teenagers' emotional well-being.

The third case study takes a systemic approach, investigating the integration of dance therapy into a larger mental health program.

This comprehensive approach stresses collaboration between mental health experts and dance therapists, acknowledging the benefits of merging established therapeutic methods with embodied movement techniques. The case study looks into logistical factors, participant experiences, and overall program success, demonstrating dance therapy's potential as a central and integrated component of comprehensive mental health interventions.

From the broader perspective, these case studies suggest that dance therapy has enormous potential as a method for emotional expression and well-being across varied communities.

Dance's embodied aspect, combined with its ability to transcend linguistic and cultural barriers, makes it an easily accessible therapy for emotional healing. As the area of mental health evolves, adopting creative and integrative techniques, dance therapy emerges as a dynamic and impactful intervention.

It encourages additional research, cooperation, and application in clinical, educational, and community contexts to fully realize its potential for increasing emotional expression and resilience. Finally, the study concludes that dance therapy is a valuable and transforming component of the overall landscape of mental health treatment, rather than a supplementary intervention.